Healing from Within:

Mastering Gut Health with a Holistic Approach

A Key to Overall Wellness

Dr. Anuj Boruah

DEDICATION

This book is dedicated to my

Respected father Late Lakhi Narayan Boruah and Loving mother Late Amiya Boruah for all the love, care, and motivation and for being the guide of my life till her death.

Second, my family, my daughter, Ansuya (Angshu), my son Ansh (Appu) and my life partner, wife Priya. Without their love, motivation, and support, it was not possible for me to complete this book.

The last one is the Health Enthusiastic readers who read this book and take action in their lives.

CONTENTS

PREFACE

Hey, Health Enthusiasts!

Ever had a gut feeling that wasn't just intuition? I did. Hi, I'm Dr. Anuj Boruah, your friendly guide to Gut Harmony. Just imagine this: bloating, discomfort, and a digestive system throwing a tantrum. Been there, felt that. That's what sparked this book—a roadmap to ditching the belly blues and reclaiming gut control!

So, why the dive into gut health? Simple. It fed me up with seeing folks struggle through digestive woes, munching on bland crackers while missing out on life's flavours. The motivation? A world where "gut issues" don't rule the roost. That's my mission.

Who's this book for? Well, anyone whose tummy plays the drums louder than a rock concert! Whether you're new to gut talk or a seasoned pro, join this gut revolution. You deserve a harmonious gut symphony, not a chaotic cacophony.

Here's the kicker: There's a treasure trove of solutions out there! But they're hidden behind bland advice and complicated jargon. Let's change that. I'm dishing out the lowdown on gut-friendly foods, lifestyle tweaks, and real, doable strategies to bring peace to your belly battleground.

Why spread the word? Because life's too short for discomfort and dietary monotony! Imagine a world where everyone savours every meal without fear of a digestive uproar. That's the utopia we're heading to, one gut at a time.

So, buckle up, dear reader. We're on a rollercoaster ride to gut wellness, sprinkled with humour, science-backed hacks, and a dash of rebel spirit. Let's turn those grumbling guts into a harmonious orchestra of health!

Cheers to gut happiness,

Dr. Anuj Boruah

INTRODUCTION

Welcome and Introduction to Gut Health

Welcome to a transformative journey towards optimal gut health! I'm delighted to introduce you to the fascinating and crucial aspect of gut health. The gut, commonly known as the digestive or gastrointestinal tract. It is a complex system composed of organs such as the mouth, esophagus, stomach, and intestines. A healthy gut is essential for overall health and well-being, as it can help boost the immune system, protect the body from harmful pathogens, improve digestion, and reduce the risk of chronic diseases such as diabetes, obesity and heart disease. Maintaining a healthy gut requires eating a balanced diet rich in fiber, staying hydrated, avoiding processed foods, and getting enough sleep. Problems with gut health can lead to various digestive disorders such as irritable bowel syndrome, inflammatory bowel disease, and celiac disease, etc. etc.

In this comprehensive guide, we begin a journey of exploration to the intricate world of gut harmony and its profound impact on our overall well-being.

Your gut is far more than a mere digestive system; it is an intricate ecosystem teeming with trillions of microorganisms that play a pivotal role in your health. From your immune function to your mood and energy levels, the health of your gut holds the key to several aspects of your life.

I planned this guide to be your compass, navigating thru the complex terrain of gut health. We will delve into the fascinating realm of the gut microbiome, unravelling its mysteries and understanding how it influences our physical and mental health.

Understanding the factors that affect gut health and learning to make informed choices regarding nutrition, lifestyle, and holistic well-being is central to this journey. Here, you'll discover applicable, evidence-based strategies and practical tips to nurture and optimize your gut health.

Our aim is simple yet profound: to empower you with the knowledge and tools necessary to cultivate a harmonious relationship with your gut. By implementing the guidance within these pages, you'll embark on a transformative path toward vitality, resilience, and overall wellness.

So, let's embark on this enlightening expedition together, as we uncover the secrets to achieving Gut Harmony!

The Importance of Gut Health in Overall Well-being

Your gut health isn't just about digestion; it's a cornerstone of your overall well-being. The gut plays a pivotal role far beyond breaking down food—it acts as a central hub influencing various bodily functions and systems.

Microbiome Mastery: At the heart of gut health lies the microbiome, an intricate ecosystem of bacteria, viruses, and fungi. This community of microorganisms living in your gut doesn't just aid digestion; it influences your immune system, metabolism, mental health, and more. A balanced and diverse microbiome is crucial for maintaining optimal health.

Immune Function: Did you know that around 70% of your immune system lives in your gut? A healthy gut microbiome helps regulate immune responses, warding off infections, allergies, and inflammation.

Mood and Brain Health: The gut-brain connection, often referred to as the "gut-brain axis," showcases the strong link between gut health and mental well-being. The microbiome produces neurotransmitters like serotonin, affecting mood, stress levels, and cognitive function.

Nutrient Absorption: A functioning gut ensures efficient absorption of nutrients from the food you eat. This absorption is critical for providing your body with essential vitamins, minerals, and energy for daily activities.

Disease Prevention: Research links an imbalance in gut health to various health issues, including obesity, diabetes, autoimmune diseases, and even certain mental health disorders. Maintaining gut harmony contributes to disease prevention and management.

Understanding the profound impact of gut health on your overall well-being is the first step toward nurturing and optimizing this vital system. The choices you make regarding nutrition, lifestyle, and self-care influence the health of your gut, paving the way for a healthier, happier you.

CHAPTER 1

Understanding Gut Health

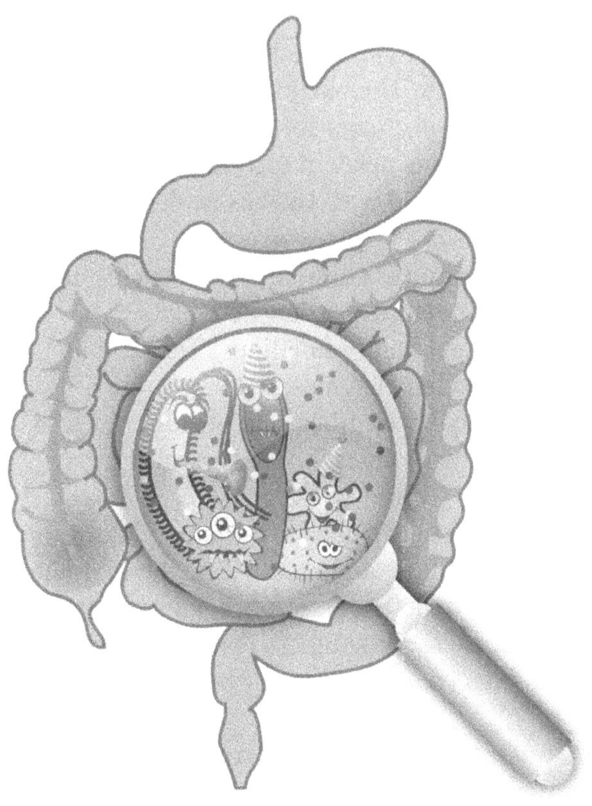

Exploring the Gut Microbiome

The gut microbiome, an intricate and diverse ecosystem of microorganisms live in your digestive tract, is an astonishingly complex and dynamic entity. Comprising trillions of bacteria, viruses, fungi, and other microbes, this bustling community forms a symbiotic relationship with our bodies, exerting a profound influence on our health.

Diversity and Balance: A healthy gut microbiome thrives on diversity. The balance between different microbial species is crucial for optimal gut function. When this balance is upset, it can lead to dysbiosis—a condition associated with various health issues.

Microbial Functions: These microorganisms aren't merely passive inhabitants; they actively get involved in crucial bodily functions. They aid in digestion, producing enzymes that break down complex carbohydrates, fiber, and other compounds that our bodies can't digest on their own.

Immune Support: The gut microbiome plays a pivotal role in training and modulating the immune system. Certain beneficial microbes help regulate immune responses, while others compete with harmful pathogens, bolstering our body's defences.

Neurotransmitter Production: Amazingly, the gut microbiome produces neurotransmitters like

Serotonin often referred to as the "happy hormone." These compounds influence mood, stress levels, and cognitive function, highlighting the strong gut-brain connection.

Factors Influencing the Microbiome: Diet, lifestyle, medications, stress, and environmental factors profoundly affect the composition and diversity of the gut microbiome. Making informed choices about nutrition and lifestyle can significantly influence the health of this microbial community.

Understanding the intricacies of the gut microbiome is pivotal in appreciating its role in our overall well-being. Nurturing a diverse and balanced microbiome through dietary choices, probiotics, prebiotics, and lifestyle modifications is fundamental to fostering gut harmony and optimal health.

Factors Affecting Gut Health

1. **Dietary Choices:** The food we consume directly influences the composition and diversity of our gut microbiome. Diets high in fiber, diverse plant-based foods, and fermented products nourish beneficial gut bacteria. Conversely, diets rich in processed foods, high sugar, and low fiber content can disrupt the microbial balance, affecting gut health.

2. **Stress and Mental Health:** The gut-brain axis connects the central nervous system to the gut,

showcasing the bidirectional communication between the two. Stress, anxiety, and other mental health issues can affect gut health by altering the gut microbiota composition, leading to digestive issues and immune system imbalances.

3. **Medications and antibiotics:** Certain medications, especially antibiotics, can indiscriminately disrupt the gut microbiome by eliminating both harmful and beneficial bacteria. Prolonged or frequent use of antibiotics can lead to dysbiosis, affecting gut health and overall well-being.

4. **Lifestyle Factors:** Sedentary lifestyles and inadequate physical activity can affect gut motility, leading to constipation or other digestive issues. Conversely, regular exercise promotes gut health by enhancing microbial diversity and metabolic function.

5. **Environmental Factors:** Exposure to environmental toxins, pollutants, and certain chemicals can influence gut health. Likewise, factors like pollution and the quality of drinking water can indirectly affect the gut microbiome.

6. **Sleep Patterns:** Disrupted sleep patterns or insufficient sleep can affect gut health. Poor sleep can alter the gut microbiota and impair digestive

processes, potentially leading to inflammation and other gut-related issues.

Understanding these various factors that influence gut health empowers individuals to make informed choices to support a healthy gut. Implementing strategies to mitigate negative influences and prioritize habits that promote gut harmony can significantly enhance overall well-being.

The Gut-Brain Connection

It intricately linked the gut and the brain through a complex communication network known as the gut-brain axis. This bidirectional pathway facilitates constant communication between the central nervous system and the enteric nervous system of the gut, influencing various physiological and psychological processes.

Neurotransmitter Production: The gut produces an array of neurotransmitters, including serotonin, dopamine, and gamma-aminobutyric acid (GABA). Serotonin, in particular, often referred to as the "feel-good" neurotransmitter, plays a crucial role in regulating mood, sleep, appetite, and even pain perception. The gut produces approximately 90% of serotonins.

Impact on Mental Health: The gut microbiome influences the production and function of these neurotransmitters, exerting a profound impact on mental health and emotional well-being. It has linked imbalances in the gut microbiota to conditions like anxiety, depression, and stress disorders.

Stress Response: Conversely, the brain can influence gut function through stress responses. Stressful situations trigger the release of stress hormones, affecting gut motility, increasing permeability, and altering the gut microbiome composition. Chronic stress can lead to gastrointestinal issues and exacerbate pre-existing gut conditions.

Immune System Regulation: The gut-brain axis also modulates the immune system. Signals from the gut influence immune responses and inflammation levels throughout the body. Dysregulation on this axis can contribute to autoimmune conditions and inflammatory bowel diseases.

Therapeutic Implications: Understanding the gut-brain connection has led to emerging therapeutic approaches like psychobiotics—probiotics with mental health benefits—and interventions targeting gut health to alleviate certain neurological and psychological disorders.

Recognizing the profound influence of the gut-brain connection underscores the importance of maintaining gut health for overall well-being.

Strategies such as stress management, a balanced diet, probiotics, and lifestyle modifications can positively affect this intricate relationship, promoting both gut and mental health.

CHAPTER 2

Nutrition for Gut Health

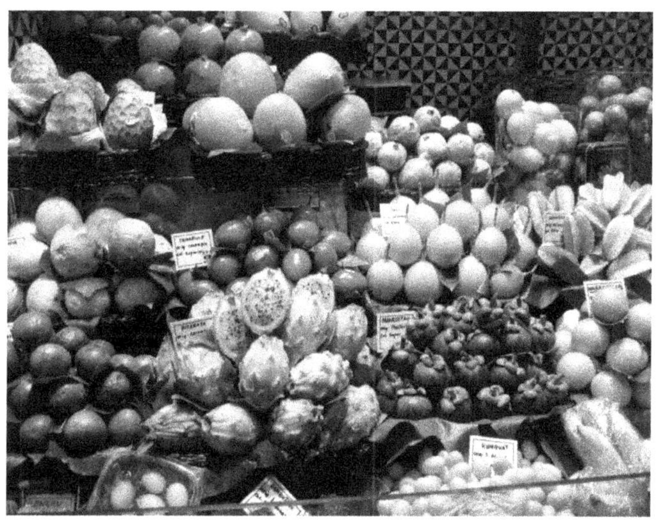

Probiotics, Prebiotics, and Their Role in Gut Health

Probiotics: Probiotics are live microorganisms—usually beneficial bacteria or yeasts—that confer health benefits when consumed in adequate amounts. These friendly microbes help maintain a healthy gut environment by fostering a balanced microbiome.

Types of Probiotics: Various strains of bacteria and yeasts fall under the probiotic umbrella, with the most common being Lactobacillus and Bifidobacterium species. As each strain may offer different health benefits, so diversity in probiotic intake is often recommended.

Functions of Probiotics:

· **Restoring Gut Balance:** Probiotics help replenish and maintain a diverse population of beneficial bacteria in the gut, preventing overgrowth of harmful microorganisms.

· **Enhancing Digestion:** They aid in breaking down food components, assisting in the digestion of certain carbohydrates and fibers that the human body can't digest alone.

· **Boosting Immune Function:** Probiotics support the immune system by promoting the production of immune-regulating compounds and enhancing the gut's defense against pathogens.

Sources of probiotics: Fermented foods like yogurt, kefir, kimchi, sauerkraut, miso, tempeh, and certain supplements contain probiotics. These sources provide a diverse range of beneficial microbes that contribute to gut health.

Prebiotics: Prebiotics are non-digestible fibers or compounds that act as food for the beneficial bacteria already present in the gut. They serve as nourishment for probiotics, stimulating their growth and activity.

Functions of Prebiotics:

· **Fuel for Beneficial Bacteria:** Prebiotics pass through the digestive tract without being digested themselves but serve as a source of nutrition for beneficial gut bacteria.

· **Supporting Gut Health:** By promoting the growth of beneficial bacteria, prebiotics help maintain a healthy balance in the gut microbiome, supporting overall digestive health and regularity.

Sources of Prebiotics: Foods rich in prebiotics include certain fruits (such as bananas, apples), vegetables (like onions, garlic), whole grains, legumes, and certain nuts and seeds. These foods contain fibers like inulin, oligofructose, and other compounds that act as prebiotics.

Synergistic Action: Probiotics and prebiotics often work together synergistically to optimize gut health. Consuming both can promote the growth and activity of beneficial gut bacteria, enhancing overall digestive wellness.

Incorporating a diverse range of probiotic-rich foods along with prebiotic sources into your diet can contribute to a flourishing gut microbiome, supporting digestive health and overall well-being.

Gut-Friendly Foods and Their Benefits

1. Fiber-Rich Foods:

· **Benefits:** Fiber is essential for gut health, as it promotes regular bowel movements and aids in the growth of beneficial gut bacteria. Soluble fiber, found in foods like oats, legumes, and fruits, forms a gel-like substance in the gut, feeding beneficial bacteria. Insoluble fiber, present in vegetables and whole grains, adds bulk to stools, aiding in their smooth passage.

· **Examples:** Berries, apples, avocados, beans, lentils, whole grains, nuts, seeds, and vegetables like broccoli and Brussels sprouts are excellent sources of fiber.

2. Fermented Foods:

· **Benefits:** Fermented foods contain live beneficial bacteria (probiotics) that support a healthy gut microbiome. These foods aid in digestion, improve nutrient absorption, and contribute to a balanced gut environment.

· **Examples:** Yogurt, kefir, kimchi, sauerkraut, miso, tempeh, and kombucha are popular fermented foods that provide a diverse range of beneficial microbes.

3. Prebiotic-Rich Foods:

· **Benefits:** Prebiotic-rich foods serve as fuel for beneficial gut bacteria, promoting their growth and activity. They contribute to a thriving gut microbiome, supporting overall digestive health.

· **Examples:** Onions, garlic, leeks, asparagus, bananas, oats, Jerusalem artichokes, and chicory root are sources of prebiotic fibers that nourish gut bacteria.

4. Polyphenol-Rich Foods:

· **Benefits:** Polyphenols are plant compounds with antioxidant properties that support gut health by reducing inflammation and promoting the growth of beneficial bacteria.

· **Examples:** Berries, dark chocolate, green tea, red grapes, flaxseeds, nuts, and certain herbs like cloves and rosemary contain high levels of polyphenols.

5. Omega-3 Fatty Acids:

· **Benefits:** Omega-3 fatty acids possess anti-inflammatory properties that contribute to a healthy gut lining, reducing the risk of gastrointestinal issues.

· **Examples:** Fatty fish (salmon, mackerel), flaxseeds, chia seeds, walnuts, and algae oil are excellent sources of omega-3 fatty acids.

6. Probiotic Supplements:

· **Benefits:** Probiotic supplements provide concentrated doses of beneficial bacteria, aiding in restoring and maintaining gut balance.

· **Examples:** Probiotic supplements containing various strains of Lactobacillus, Bifidobacterium, or Saccharomyces boulardii are available on the market.

Incorporating a diverse array of these gut-friendly foods into your diet can promote a healthy gut microbiome, supporting digestion, immune function, and overall well-being.

Foods to Avoid for a Healthy Gut

1. Highly Processed Foods:

· **Reason:** Processed foods often contain high amounts of added sugars, unhealthy fats, artificial additives, and preservatives. These can disrupt the balance of gut bacteria and contribute to inflammation in the digestive system.

· **Examples:** Packaged snacks, fast food, sugary cereals, processed meats, and ready-to-eat meals usually fall under this category.

2. Artificial Sweeteners:

· **Reason:** Some artificial sweeteners, despite being low in calories, can negatively affect gut bacteria composition and interfere with glucose metabolism, potentially leading to digestive issues.

· **Examples:** Aspartame (Equal), saccharin (Sweet'N Low), sucralose (Splenda), and sugar alcohols like sorbitol and xylitol.

3. High-Sugar Foods:

· **Reason:** Excessive sugar consumption can promote the growth of harmful bacteria in the gut and contribute to inflammation. It may also lead to conditions like small intestinal bacterial overgrowth (SIBO) and contribute to dysbiosis.

· **Examples:** Soda, candies, pastries, desserts, sweetened beverages, and foods with high sugar content.

4. Artificial Additives and Preservatives:

· **Reason:** Artificial additives and preservatives in processed foods can disrupt the gut microbiome and cause irritation to the gastrointestinal lining, potentially leading to digestive discomfort.

· **Examples:** Artificial colors, flavors, emulsifiers, and preservatives commonly found in processed and packaged foods.

5. High-Fat Foods:

· **Reason:** While healthy fats are beneficial, excessive intake of saturated and trans fats found in fried foods and certain processed items can lead to inflammation and negatively impact gut health.

· **Examples:** Deep-fried foods, fatty cuts of meat, processed foods high in trans fats, and hydrogenated oils.

6. Gluten and Certain Grains:

· **Reason:** For individuals with gluten sensitivity or celiac disease, gluten-containing grains like wheat, barley, and rye can cause inflammation, digestive discomfort, and damage to the gut lining.

· **Examples:** Wheat-based products, barley, rye, and some processed foods containing gluten derivatives.

7. Excessive Alcohol:

· **Reason:** Excessive alcohol consumption can disrupt the gut microbiome, damage the gut lining, and lead to inflammation in the gastrointestinal tract.

· **Examples:** Regular and excessive intake of alcoholic beverages.

Avoiding or minimizing these foods in your diet can contribute to a healthier gut environment, supporting optimal digestion and overall gut health.

CHAPTER 3

Personalized Nutrition Strategies

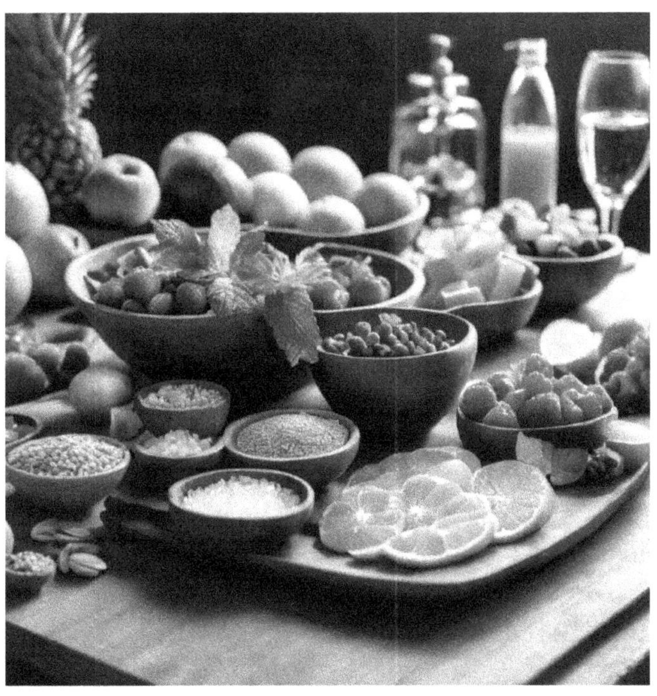

Tailoring Diet Plans for Gut Health

1. Emphasize Fiber-Rich Foods:

· **Diverse Sources:** Include a variety of fiber-rich foods such as fruits, vegetables, whole grains, legumes, nuts, and seeds. This diverse range of fibers nourishes different beneficial bacteria, promoting a healthy gut microbiome.

· **Gradual Increase:** Gradually increase fiber intake to allow the gut to adapt. Sudden drastic changes may cause temporary digestive discomfort.

2. Incorporate Probiotic Foods:

· **Diverse Strains:** Include a variety of fermented foods rich in probiotics to introduce diverse strains of beneficial bacteria into the gut. Yogurt, kefir, sauerkraut, kimchi, miso, tempeh, and kombucha are excellent choices.

· **Regular Consumption:** Incorporate probiotic-rich foods into your diet regularly to maintain a diverse and balanced gut microbiome.

3. Include Prebiotic Foods:

· **Diverse Selection:** Consume prebiotic-rich foods to support the growth and activity of beneficial gut bacteria. Onions, garlic, leeks, bananas, asparagus, oats, and legumes are valuable sources of prebiotics.

· **Varied Diet:** Aim for a varied diet that includes different prebiotic fibers to nourish a wide range of gut bacteria.

4. Limit Processed Foods and Sugars:

· **Minimize Consumption:** Reduce intake of highly processed foods, refined sugars, and artificial additives that can negatively affect gut health and disrupt the gut microbiome.

· **Read Labels:** Check food labels and avoid products with high levels of added sugars, artificial sweeteners, and preservatives.

5. Consider Gluten and FODMAPs Sensitivities:

· **Personalized Approach:** For individuals sensitive to gluten or certain carbohydrates known as FODMAPs (fermentable oligosaccharides, disaccharides, monosaccharides, and polyols), consider a diet that avoids these triggers.

· **Consultation:** Seek guidance from a healthcare professional or registered dietician to determine if a low-FODMAP or gluten-free diet is suitable for your specific needs.

6. Stay Hydrated and Mindful of Portions:

· **Adequate Hydration:** Drink plenty of water to support digestion and prevent constipation. Proper hydration helps maintain gut motility and aids in nutrient absorption.

· **Portion Control:** Practice mindful eating and portion control. Overeating can overwhelm the digestive system and lead to discomfort.

Customizing a diet plan for gut health involves a holistic approach, focusing on whole, nutrient-dense foods that promote a balanced gut microbiome and support optimal digestive function.

Meal Planning for Gut Harmony

1. Focus on Diversity:

· **Varied Food Groups:** Include a variety of foods from all food groups to ensure a diverse nutrient intake. Incorporate fruits, vegetables, whole grains, lean proteins, healthy fats, and legumes into your meals.

· **Colorful Plate:** Aim for a colorful plate, as different-colored fruits and vegetables provide various nutrients and antioxidants beneficial for gut health.

2. Balanced Macronutrients:

· **Healthy Balance:** Ensure each meal contains a balance of carbohydrates, proteins, and fats. Healthy fats from sources like avocados, nuts, seeds, and fatty fish can support gut health and overall wellness.

· **Moderate Portions:** Pay attention to portion sizes to avoid overeating, which can strain the digestive system.

3. Regular Meal Times:

· **Consistent Schedule:** Establish regular meal times to maintain a steady rhythm for digestion. Consistency in meal timing can support digestive processes and aid in nutrient absorption.

· **Mindful Eating:** Practice mindful eating, focusing on enjoying and savoring your meals without distractions, which aids in proper digestion.

4. Incorporate Gut-Friendly Foods:

· **Probiotic-Rich Choices:** Include probiotic-rich foods like yogurt, kefir, kimchi, sauerkraut, or kombucha in your meal plan to introduce beneficial bacteria into your gut.

· **Prebiotic Sources:** Incorporate prebiotic-rich foods such as onions, garlic, asparagus, bananas, oats, and legumes to nourish the beneficial gut bacteria.

5. Plan Preparations Mindfully:

· **Gentle Cooking Methods:** Use gentle cooking techniques like steaming, boiling, or baking rather than heavy frying, which may strip nutrients and add unnecessary fats.

· **Homemade Meals:** Opt for homemade meals to have better control over ingredients and avoid excessive additives or preservatives.

6. Hydration and Herbal Teas:

· **Adequate Water Intake:** Stay hydrated by drinking sufficient water throughout the day. Herbal teas like peppermint or ginger tea can also support digestion.

· **Limit Stimulants:** Minimize or avoid excessive consumption of caffeinated or sugary beverages that might irritate the gut lining.

7. Plan and Prepare Ahead:

· **Weekly Planning:** Plan meals for the week ahead to ensure a well-rounded and gut-supportive diet.

Preparing meals ahead of time can facilitate healthier eating habits.

· **Batch Cooking:** Consider batch cooking or preparing components of meals in advance to save time and ensure healthier choices are readily available.

Meal planning for gut harmony involves thoughtful consideration of foods that support a healthy gut microbiome while maintaining a balanced and enjoyable diet. Tailor your meals to your preferences, dietary needs, and individual gut health goals.

Creating a Balanced Gut Ecosystem

1. Embrace a Diverse Diet:

· **Variety of Foods:** Aim for a diverse diet rich in fruits, vegetables, whole grains, lean proteins, nuts, seeds, and legumes. Fresh foods nourish the beneficial bacteria, promoting a diverse gut microbiome.

· **Include Prebiotics:** Incorporate prebiotic-rich foods like onions, garlic, asparagus, bananas, oats, and legumes to provide nourishment for beneficial gut bacteria.

2. Probiotics for Gut Health:

· **Fermented Foods:** Regularly consume fermented foods rich in probiotics, such as yogurt, kefir, kimchi, sauerkraut, miso, tempeh, and kombucha. These foods introduce beneficial bacteria into the gut.

· **Consider Supplements:** In some cases, probiotic supplements may be beneficial, especially after a course of antibiotics or for specific gut health issues. Consult a healthcare professional for guidance.

3. Avoid Excessive Antibiotics:

· **Selective Use:** Minimize unnecessary or excessive antibiotic use if not essential. Antibiotics can disrupt the gut microbiome by indiscriminately killing both harmful and beneficial bacteria.

· **Post-Antibiotic Care:** If antibiotics are necessary, consider post-antibiotic care, including probiotic supplementation and focus on prebiotic-rich foods to restore gut balance.

4. Manage Stress Levels:

· **Stress Reduction Techniques:** Practice stress management techniques like meditation, yoga, deep breathing exercises, or mindfulness practices. Chronic stress can negatively affect the gut microbiome and digestive health.

· **Regular Exercise:** Engage in regular physical activity as it can positively influence gut health by promoting a more diverse microbiome.

5. Adequate Sleep and Hydration:

· **Quality Sleep:** Prioritize adequate sleep as insufficient sleep can disrupt the gut microbiota and impact overall health. Aim for 7-9 hours of quality sleep each night.

· **Hydration:** Stay well-hydrated by drinking plenty of water. Proper hydration supports digestion and maintains gut motility.

6. Minimize Processed Foods and Sugars:

· **Limit Highly Processed Foods:** Reduce intake of processed foods high in added sugars, unhealthy fats, and artificial additives. These can negatively affect the gut microbiome and contribute to inflammation.

· **Moderate Sugar Intake:** Minimize consumption of refined sugars and artificial sweeteners, which may disturb gut health and exacerbate certain digestive issues.

7. Consistency in Habits:

· **Regular Eating Patterns:** Aim for consistent meal times and eating patterns to support a healthy gut environment. Regularity helps in maintaining a balanced gut ecosystem.

· **Gradual Changes:** Implement dietary changes gradually to allow the gut microbiome time to adapt and avoid potential digestive discomfort.

Cultivating a balanced gut ecosystem involves a holistic approach, focusing on dietary diversity, probiotics, stress management, adequate sleep, and hydration. Small, consistent lifestyle changes can positively affect gut health in daily life.

CHAPTER 4

Lifestyle Factors Impacting Gut Health

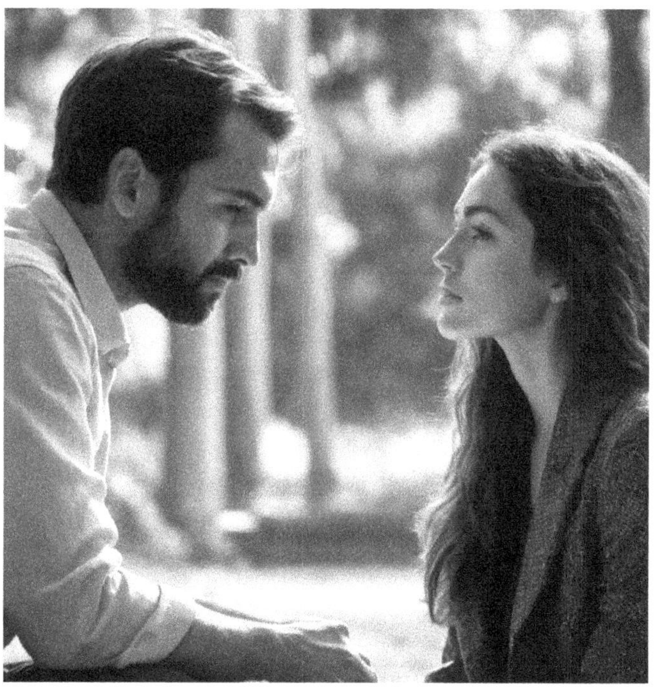

Stress Management Techniques

1. Mindfulness Meditation:

· **Practice Focus:** Mindfulness meditation involves focusing on the present moment without judgment. It helps reduce stress by promoting relaxation and increasing self-awareness.

· **Technique:** Find a quiet space, sit comfortably, and focus on your breath or a specific sensation. When thoughts arise, gently bring your attention back to the present moment.

2. Deep Breathing Exercises:

· **Diaphragmatic Breathing:** Deep breathing techniques, such as diaphragmatic breathing or belly breathing, promote relaxation and reduce stress. It involves inhaling deeply through the nose, allowing the belly to rise, and exhaling slowly through the mouth.

· **Regular Practice:** Practice deep breathing exercises regularly, especially during stressful moments or as part of a daily relaxation routine.

3. Progressive Muscle Relaxation (PMR):

· **Muscle Relaxation:** PMR involves systematically tensing and then relaxing different muscle groups in the body. It helps release physical tension and promotes relaxation.

· **Step-by-Step Approach:** Start by tensing and relaxing each muscle group, progressing from your toes to your head, focusing on each group for several seconds before moving on.

4. Yoga and Tai Chi:

· **Mind-Body Connection:** Yoga and Tai Chi combine movement, breathwork, and mindfulness, promoting relaxation and reducing stress. These practices improve flexibility, balance, and overall well-being.

· **Regular Practice:** Engage in yoga or Tai Chi classes or follow guided sessions to experience their stress-relieving benefits.

5. Exercise and Physical Activity:

· **Stress-Reducing Effects:** Regular physical activity, such as walking, running, dancing, aerobics or zumba can help reduce stress and anxiety by releasing endorphins, the body's natural mood lifters.

· **Consistent Routine:** Establish a routine that includes regular exercise to benefit both physical and mental health.

6. Mindfulness-Based Stress Reduction (MBSR):

· **Structured Program:** MBSR is an evidence-based program that combines mindfulness meditation and yoga to reduce stress. It teaches techniques to cope with stress and enhance self-awareness.

· **Participation:** Consider enrolling in an MBSR program or accessing online resources that offer structured guidance in stress reduction techniques.

7. Relaxation Techniques and Hobbies:

· **Creative Outlets:** Engaging in hobbies or activities that bring joy, such as painting, gardening, playing music, or reading, can reduce stress and promote relaxation.

· **Prioritize Relaxation:** Dedicate time for activities that relax and rejuvenate you, balancing work or other stress-inducing responsibilities.

Incorporating these stress management techniques into daily life can significantly reduce stress levels, promote relaxation, and positively impact overall health, including gut health.

Explore and incorporate these techniques into your routine, adjusting them to suit your preferences and lifestyle for optimal stress management!

Exercise and Its Effect on Gut Health

1. Improved Gut Motility:

· **Enhanced Digestion:** Regular physical activity promotes gut motility, aiding in the movement of food through the digestive tract. This helps prevent issues like constipation and supports regular bowel movements.

2. Modulation of Gut Microbiota:

· **Increased Microbial Diversity:** It linked Exercise to a more diverse gut microbiota, promoting a healthier balance of beneficial bacteria. This diversity is associated with better overall gut health.

· **Impact on Microbial Composition:** Studies suggest that exercise can alter the composition and abundance of gut bacteria, contributing to a more favourable gut environment.

3. Reduction of inflammation:

· **Anti-Inflammatory Effects:** Physical activity helps reduce systemic inflammation, which can positively affect gut health. It linked chronic inflammation in the gut to various digestive disorders.

4. Stress Reduction and Gut Health:

· **Stress Management:** Exercise can reduce stress and anxiety levels, which is indirectly benefited our gut health. Lower stress levels are associated with a healthier gut environment.

· **Mind-Body Connection:** Improved mental health through exercise can positively influence the gut-brain axis, affecting gut function and overall well-being.

5. Regulation of Immune Function:

· **Enhanced Immune Response:** Moderate exercise supports a robust immune system, which indirectly affects gut health. A balanced immune response is crucial for maintaining gut integrity and health.

6. Weight Management and Gut Health:

· **Weight Regulation:** Regular exercise plays a role in weight management, and maintaining a healthy weight can positively affect gut health. Obesity is linked to gut dysbiosis and increased gut-related issues.

7. Timing and Type of Exercise:

· **Consistency Matters:** Consistent, moderate exercise is more beneficial for gut health than sporadic or intense workouts. Finding a routine that suits your lifestyle is key.

· **Varied Activities:** While any exercise is beneficial, a combination of aerobic activities (like walking, jogging, cycling, or zumba) and strength training can offer comprehensive health benefits, including for gut health.

8. Hydration and Exercise:

· **Proper Hydration:** Staying hydrated is crucial during exercise as it supports proper digestion and overall guts function. Maintain adequate fluid intake before, during, and after physical activity.

Incorporating regular exercise into your routine offers lots of benefits beyond physical fitness, positively affecting gut health by supporting digestion, modulating the gut microbiota, reducing inflammation, and managing stress levels.

Always consult with a healthcare professional before making some changes to your exercise routine, especially if you have existing health conditions.

Sleep and Its Influence on Digestion

1. Gut Motility and Regularity:

· **Regulated Digestive Process:** During sleep, the body continues its digestive functions, albeit at a slower pace. Adequate sleep supports proper gut motility and allows for the efficient movement of food through the digestive tract.

· **Healthy Bowel Movements:** Consistent and restful sleep patterns contribute to regular bowel movements, promoting overall digestive regularity.

2. Gut Microbiome and Sleep:

· **Microbial Balance:** Sleep plays a role in maintaining a healthy balance of gut microbes. Disrupted sleep patterns or insufficient sleep may affect the diversity and composition of gut bacteria, potentially affecting digestion.

· **Bidirectional Relationship:** The gut microbiome can also influence sleep patterns via the gut-brain axis, affecting sleep quality and duration.

3. Hormonal Regulation:

· **Appetite Hormones:** Sleep deprivation can disrupt the balance of appetite-regulating hormones such as leptin and ghrelin. This imbalance might lead to altered hunger cues, potentially affecting food choices and digestion.

· **Insulin Sensitivity:** Inadequate sleep can affect insulin sensitivity, potentially contributing to changes in metabolism and digestion.

4. Gut-Brain Axis and Sleep:

· **Impact on Mood and Stress:** Quality sleep supports mental health and reduces stress levels, which positively affects gut health. Disrupted sleep patterns can affect mood and stress responses, potentially affecting digestive processes.

· **Stress and Digestion:** Poor sleep quality may increase stress hormones like cortisol, which can affect gut permeability and contribute to digestive discomfort.

5. Circadian Rhythm and Digestive Functions:

· **Synchronized Functions:** The body's internal clock, or circadian rhythm, influences digestive functions. Regular sleeps patterns help synchronize this rhythm, optimizing digestion and nutrient absorption.

· **Meal Timing:** Consistent sleep schedules positively impact meal timing, allowing the body to take action in preparation digestive processes more effectively.

6. Digestive Disorders and Sleep:

· **Reciprocal Relationship:** Conditions like gastroesophageal reflux disease (GERD), irritable bowel syndrome (IBS), or inflammatory bowel disease (IBD) can affect sleep quality due to discomfort to symptoms.

· **Managing Both:** Improving sleep quality and patterns can sometimes reduces symptoms of digestive disorders, while managing digestive issues can lead to better sleep.

7. Hydration and Bedtime Habits:

· **Hydration Practices:** Maintaining proper hydration throughout the day supports digestive functions, but it's advisable to avoid excessive fluids close to bedtime to prevent disruptions due to frequent bathroom visits.

· **Pre-Sleep Routines:** Establishing relaxing pre-sleep routines, such as gentle stretches, reading, or taking a warm bath, can contribute to better sleep quality and indirectly support digestion.

Prioritizing regular, restful sleep is essential for overall health, including optimal digestion. Aiming for consistent sleep schedules and healthy sleep habits contributes to a balanced digestive system and improved gastrointestinal well-being.

Consult with a healthcare professional if you have persistent digestive issues or sleep disturbances affecting your health.

CHAPTER 5

Recipes for Gut-Friendly Meals

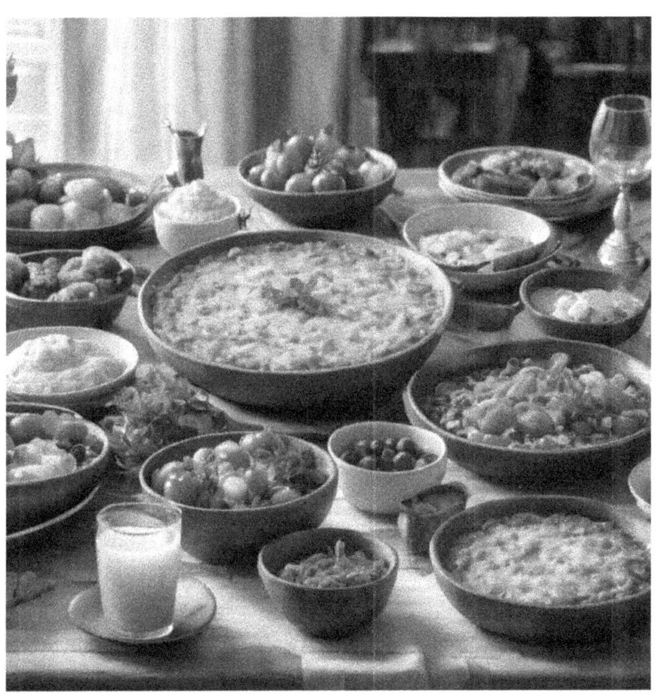

Recipes Supporting Gut Health

1. Greek Yogurt Parfait:

· **Ingredients:**

· Greek yogurt (probiotic-rich)

· Berries (blueberries, strawberries)

· Chia seeds (source of fiber)

· Honey or maple syrup (optional for sweetness)

· **Preparation:** Layer Greek yogurt with berries and chia seeds in a glass, drizzle with honey or maple syrup. Enjoy as a nutrient-packed breakfast or snack.

2. Quinoa and Veggie Buddha Bowl:

· **Ingredients:**

· Cooked quinoa (source of prebiotics)

· Mixed vegetables (bell peppers, kale, broccoli)

· Chickpeas (fiber-rich legumes)

· Avocado slices (healthy fats)

· Lemon-tahini dressing

· **Preparation:** Arrange cooked quinoa, roasted vegetables, chickpeas, and avocado in a bowl. Drizzle with lemon-tahini dressing for a flavorful and gut-nourishing meal.

3. Miso-Glazed Salmon:

· **Ingredients:**

· Salmon fillets (source of omega-3 fatty acids)

· Miso paste (probiotic-rich)

· Soy sauce or tamari

· Garlic and ginger (for flavor)

· **Preparation:** Mix miso paste, soy sauce, garlic, and ginger. Coat salmon fillets and bake or grill until cooked through. Serve with steamed vegetables for a gut-supporting dinner.

4. Lentil and Vegetable Soup:

· **Ingredients:**

· Lentils (high in fiber and protein)

· Carrots, celery, onions, and spinach

· Vegetable broth

· Turmeric and cumin (anti-inflammatory spices)

· **Preparation:** Sauté vegetables, add lentils, broth, and spices. Simmer until lentils are tender. We packed this hearty soup with gut-friendly nutrients.

5. Kimchi Fried Rice:

· **Ingredients:**

· Cooked brown rice (source of fiber)

· Kimchi (fermented food, probiotic-rich)

· Mixed vegetables (peas, carrots, bell peppers)

· Tofu or eggs for protein (optional)

· **Preparation:** Stir-fry cooked rice with chopped kimchi, mixed vegetables, and tofu or eggs for a flavorful and gut-boosting meal.

6. Berry and Spinach Smoothie:

· **Ingredients:**

· Spinach (rich in antioxidants)

· Mixed berries (antioxidant-rich fruits)

· Kefir or yogurt (probiotic-rich)

· Chia seeds (fiber and omega-3s)

· **Preparation:** Blend spinach, berries, kefir or yogurt, and chia seeds until smooth for a refreshing and gut-nourishing smoothie.

7. Ginger-Turmeric Tea:

· **Ingredients:**

· Fresh ginger and turmeric (anti-inflammatory)

· Lemon (vitamin C)

· Honey (optional for sweetness)

· **Preparation:** Simmer sliced ginger and turmeric in water, strain, and add lemon and honey for a soothing tea to support digestion.

These recipes incorporate ingredients known for their positive impact on gut health, providing a variety of flavours and nutrients to promote a healthy digestive system.

Adjust these recipes according to dietary preferences or specific gut health needs while ensuring a balanced and nutritious diet.

Meal Ideas and Preparation Tips

1. Breakfast Ideas:

· **Overnight Oats:** Prepare oats with milk or yogurt, chia seeds, and fruits the night before for a quick and nutritious breakfast.

· **Egg and Veggie Scramble:** Sautee vegetables with eggs or tofu for a protein-packed morning meal.

· **Smoothie Bowls:** Blend greens, fruits, yogurt or kefir, and toppings like nuts or seeds for a refreshing breakfast option.

2. Lunch Ideas:

· **Salad Jars:** Layer mixed greens, veggies, beans, quinoa, or proteins in a jar for a portable and customizable salad.

· **Wraps or Sandwiches:** Use whole-grain wraps or bread with lean proteins, veggies, and health spreads like hummus or avocado.

· **Grain Bowls:** Combine cooked grains, roasted vegetables, protein (chicken, tofu), and a flavourful sauce for a satisfying lunch option.

3. Dinner Ideas:

· **Stir-Fry:** Cook lean protein with assorted vegetables and a flavorful sauce, served over brown rice or quinoa.

· **Baked Fish or Tofu:** Season fish fillets or tofu. Bake with vegetables for a simple and healthy dinner.

· **Vegetarian Chili or Soup:** Use beans, lentils, veggies, and spices for a hearty and nutritious meal.

4. Preparation Tips:

· **Batch Cooking:** Prepare ingredients in bulk for the week ahead, such as roasted veggies, cooked grains, or proteins, for quick meal assembly.

· **Meal Prepping Containers:** Use meal prep containers to portion out meals, making it easier to grab and go during busy days. Always prefer to use multilayer stainless steel cooking containers to avoid metal contaminations.

· **Smart Cooking Techniques:** Opt for healthier cooking methods like grilling, baking, steaming, or sautéing with minimal oil to keep nutrients. Low heat cooking in a multilayer stainless steel container including lid is the best to keep nutrients in the cooked food.

5. Snack Ideas:

· **Yogurt with Berries:** Greek yogurt with fresh or frozen berries provides protein and probiotics.

· **Nuts and Seeds:** A handful of nuts or seeds (almonds, walnuts, chia seeds) offer healthy fats and fibers.

· **Veggies with Hummus:** Sliced vegetables paired with hummus make a nutritious and satisfying snack.

6. Mindful Eating Tips:

· **Portion Control:** Use smaller plates and bowls to control portion sizes and avoid overeating.

· **Eat Slowly:** Chew food thoroughly and eat slowly to aid digestion and recognize fullness cues.

· **Mindful Mealtime:** Minimize distractions while eating, focusing on the flavours and textures of the food.

7. Hydration Habits:

· **Water Intake:** Keep a water bottle handy and sip throughout the day to stay adequately hydrated.

· **Herbal Teas:** Incorporate soothing herbal teas like chamomile or peppermint for hydration and relaxation.

8. Grocery Shopping Tips:

· **Fresh Produce:** Prioritize fresh fruits, vegetables, leafy greens, and colourful fruits and vegetables for a nutrient-dense diet.

· **Whole Grains:** Choose whole-grain options like brown rice, quinoa, oats, and whole-grain bread for fiber and nutrients.

· **Lean Proteins:** Opt for lean meats, fish, poultry, tofu, legumes, and beans as sources of protein.

By incorporating these meal ideas and preparation tips into your routine, you can create a diverse, nutritious, and gut-friendly diet that supports overall health and well-being.

Adapt these ideas to suit dietary preferences or specific nutritional needs while focusing on a balanced and wholesome approach to eating!

CHAPTER 6

Supplements and Gut Health

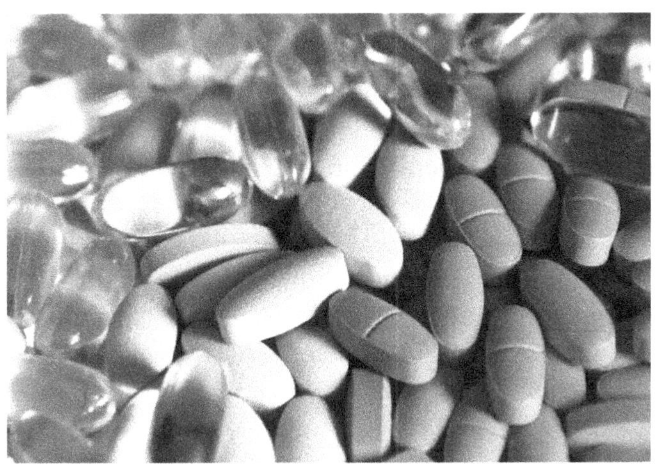

Understanding Supplements for Gut Health

1. Probiotics:

· **Function:** Probiotics are live beneficial bacteria that promote a healthy gut microbiome. They aid digestion, support immune function, and to relieve certain digestive issues.

· **Types:** Look for diverse strains like Lactobacillus and Bifidobacterium species. Consider specific strains targeting your concerns, such as L. acidophilus for lactose intolerance or B. infantis for IBS.

· **Dosage and Timing:** Follow recommended dosages and storage instructions. Some may require refrigeration. Take consistently, ideally on an empty stomach or as directed.

2. Prebiotics:

· **Function:** Prebiotics are fiber compounds that nourish and support the growth of beneficial gut bacteria. They aid in maintaining a healthy gut environment and promoting the growth of probiotics.

· **Sources:** Natural sources include garlic, onions, bananas, asparagus, oats, and Jerusalem artichokes. Prebiotic supplements may contain fibers like inulin or oligosaccharides.

3. Digestive Enzymes:

· **Function:** Digestive enzymes assist in break down macronutrients (carbohydrates, proteins, fats) for better absorption and digestion. They may help relieve symptoms of digestive issues like bloating or discomfort.

· **Types:** Common enzymes include amylase (for carbs), protease (for proteins), and lipase (for fats). Blend formulations or single enzymes are available depending on needs.

4. Fiber Supplements:

· **Function:** Fiber supplements aid in regular bowel movements, support digestive health, and feed beneficial gut bacteria. It relieves constipation or promotes overall gut motility.

· **Types:** Soluble (psyllium husk, glucomannan) and insoluble (wheat bran, cellulose) fibers. Start with lower doses and gradually increase while ensuring adequate hydration.

5. Omega-3 Fatty Acids:

· **Function:** Omega-3s possess anti-inflammatory properties beneficial for gut health. They support the gut lining, reduce inflammation, and may benefit conditions like Crohn's disease or ulcerative colitis.

· **Sources:** Supplements often contain fish oil, algae-based DHA/EPA for vegetarians/vegans. Ensure quality and purity when selecting omega-3 supplements.

6. L-Glutamine:

· **Function:** L-Glutamine is an amino acid crucial for intestinal health, aiding in gut lining repair and maintenance. It may assist in conditions like leaky gut syndrome (LGS) or intestinal inflammation.

· **Usage:** Often available as a powdered supplement. Consult a healthcare provider for proper dosage and usage guidelines.

7. Vitamin D:

· **Function:** Vitamin D plays a role in maintaining a healthy immune system and gut function. Deficiency may affect gut health and contribute to inflammatory bowel diseases.

· **Sources:** Supplements or exposure to sunlight. Opt for D3 supplements for better absorption.

8. Considerations and Recommendations:

· **Consultation:** Prioritize professional advice before starting any new supplements, especially if dealing with specific gut conditions or undergoing medical treatments.

· **Quality and Brand:** Choose reputable brands with third-party testing for quality and efficacy. Check for allergens, additives, or fillers in supplements.

· **Balanced Approach:** Supplements should complement a healthy diet, lifestyle, and potentially prescribed treatments rather than replace them.

Remember, while supplements can support gut health, they work best when integrated into a holistic approach that includes a healthy diet, regular exercise, adequate sleep, and stress management.

Always consult with a healthcare professional or a registered dietician before starting any new supplements, especially if you have existing health conditions or concerns.

Recommendations and Considerations for Gut Health Supplements

1. Professional Guidance:

· **Consult Healthcare Provider:** Before starting any new supplements, especially if managing specific gut conditions or undergoing medical treatments, consult a healthcare provider or a registered dietician.

· **Individualized Approach:** Seek personalized recommendations based on your health status, dietary habits, and potential interactions with medications or existing conditions.

2. Quality and Reliability:

· **Reputable Brands:** Choose supplements from reputable brands that adhere to Good Manufacturing Practices (GMP) and undergo third-party testing for purity and potency.

· **Check Labels:** Look for certifications, quality seals, and transparent labelling inform absence of contaminants, allergens, or unnecessary additives.

3. Types of Supplements:

· **Specific Strains and Types:** When choosing probiotics, consider the specific strains and types that target your concerns (e.g., lactose intolerance, IBS, or immune support). Different strains offer unique benefits.

· **Formulations and varieties:** Supplements come in various forms—capsules, powders, or liquids. Select the form that suits your preferences and ease of use.

4. Dosage and Usage:

· **Follow Recommendations:** Adhere to recommended dosages provided by healthcare professionals or on the supplement labels. Avoid exceeding recommended doses without guidance.

· **Timing and Consistency:** Some supplements, like probiotics or enzymes, may require specific timing (e.g., with or without food) or consistency in consumption for optimal effectiveness.

5. Individual Needs and Conditions:

· **Personalized Approach:** Consider individual needs, dietary preferences, and any pre-existing conditions when selecting supplements. Certain conditions may benefit from specific supplements, while others may require caution.

· **Potential Interactions:** Be mindful of potential interactions between supplements and medications. Some supplements may interfere with certain medications or medical conditions.

6. Lifestyle Factors:

· **Supportive Lifestyle Changes:** Supplements work best when integrated into a holistic approach that includes a balanced diet rich in fiber, whole foods, regular exercise, stress management, and adequate sleep.

· **Healthy Habits:** Supplements should complement a healthy lifestyle rather than substitute for poor dietary choices or unhealthy habits.

7. Monitor and Assess:

· **Observing Changes:** Pay attention to any changes in symptoms, digestion, or overall well-being after starting supplements. Monitor how your body responds and adjusts as necessary.

· **Reassess Periodically:** Reevaluate supplements use periodically, especially if there are changes in health status or dietary habits.

8. Consideration of Risks and Side Effects:

· **Potential Risks:** Be aware of potential risks or side effects associated with certain supplements, especially if taken in high doses or for extended periods. Report any adverse effects to healthcare professionals.

· **Balanced Approach:** Balance the potential benefits of supplements with the need to minimize risks, ensure to use safely and responsibly.

9. Long-Term Sustainability:

· **Sustainable Practices:** Aim for a sustainable and manageable supplement routine. Evaluate the long-term sustainability of supplement usage and its integration into your daily routine.

· Remember, we mean supplement to a complement of healthy lifestyle and dietary choices. It should be a part of a comprehensive approach to gut health that includes a balanced diet, exercise, adequate sleep, stress management, and professional guidance.

· Always consult with a healthcare professional or a registered dietician before initiating or changing any supplement regimen, especially if dealing with specific health concerns or conditions.

Maintaining Gut Health in the Long Term

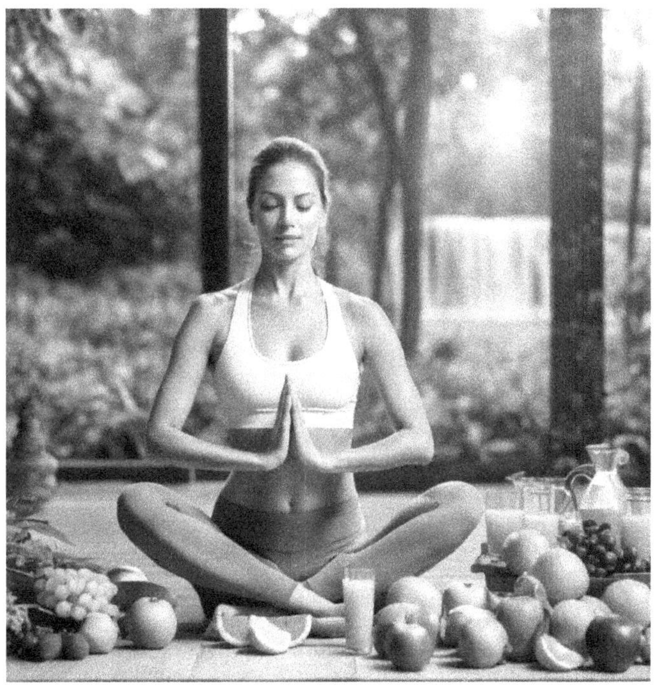

Sustaining Gut Health Beyond Diet

1. Stress Management:

· **Mindfulness Practices:** Engage in activities like meditation, deep breathing exercises, yoga, or tai chi to manage stress levels. Chronic stress can affect gut health through the gut-brain axis.

· **Regular Exercise:** Physical activity helps reduce stress hormones and promotes a healthier gut microbiome. Regular workouts contribute to overall well-being, including gut health.

2. Quality Sleep:

· **Consistent Sleep Patterns:** Prioritize sufficient sleep and aim for consistent sleep schedules. Quality sleep supports the gut microbiome, aids digestion, and regulates appetite.

· **Sleep Hygiene:** Create a conducive sleep environment by minimizing distractions, avoiding screens before bedtime, and establishing a calming bedtime routine.

3. Hydration Habits:

· **Adequate Water Intake:** Stay hydrated by consuming enough water throughout the day. Proper hydration supports digestion, nutrient absorption, and a healthy gut environment.

· **Herbal Teas:** Incorporate herbal teas like chamomile, ginger, or peppermint, known for their soothing effects on the digestive system.

4. Regular Physical Activity:

· **Moderate Exercise:** Engage in regular physical activity, which aids in maintaining a diverse gut microbiota and supports gut motility. Aim for a mix of aerobic and strength-training exercises.

· **Outdoor Activities:** Spending time outdoors and in natural environments can positively affect gut health by increasing microbial diversity.

5. Avoidance of Harmful Substances:

· **Limit Alcohol and Tobacco:** Excessive alcohol consumption and tobacco use can disrupt the gut microbiome and lead to gastrointestinal issues. Moderation or avoidance is key.

· **Minimize Antibiotics:** Use antibiotics judiciously, as they can disturb the gut microbiota. Discuss alternatives or probiotic supplementation with a healthcare professional when prescribed antibiotics.

6. Proper Medication Use:

· **Careful Use of Medications:** Be mindful of medications that may affect gut health. Discuss potential side effects with healthcare providers and consider probiotics if needed during medication courses.

· **Compliance with prescriptions:** Follow prescribed medications as directed to avoid complications that may affect gut health.

7. Gut-Friendly Habits:

· **Regular Health Check-ups:** Regular visits to healthcare providers for check-ups can identify and address any potential gut health issues early.

· **Mindful Eating:** Practice mindful eating, focusing on chewing thoroughly, eat slowly and savoring the meals. This aids digestion and nutrient absorption.

8. Psychological Well-being:

· **Positive Social Connections:** Cultivate healthy social relationships and meaningful connections, as social interactions can positively affect mental health and indirectly support gut health.

· **Seeking Support:** Address emotional well-being by seeking professional support if dealing with chronic stress, anxiety, or other mental health concerns.

9. Environmental Factors:

· **Limit Exposure to toxins:** Minimize exposure to environmental toxins and pollutants, which can affect gut health and overall well-being.

· **Healthy Home Environment:** Ensure a hygiene and clean living space to minimize exposure to harmful substances.

Sustaining gut health involves a holistic approach that encompasses various lifestyle factors beyond dietary choices. Prioritizing stress management, quality sleep, regular exercise, and a healthy lifestyle contributes to a balanced and thriving gut environment.

Incorporating these practices into daily life can significantly contribute to maintaining optimal gut health and overall well-being.

Habits and Practices for Ongoing Wellness

1. Physical Wellness:

· **Regular Exercise Routine:** Engage in a mix of cardiovascular, strength training, and flexibility exercises for overall physical fitness.

· **Prioritize Movement:** Incorporate physical activity into daily routines, such as walking, taking the stairs, or stretching breaks throughout the day.

· **Adequate Rest and Recovery:** Balance workouts with sufficient rest and recovery to prevent injuries and support overall well-being.

2. Nutrition and Diet:

· **Balanced Diet:** Focus on whole foods, fruits, vegetables, lean proteins, healthy fats, and complex carbohydrates for a nutrient-rich diet.

· **Mindful Eating:** Pay attention to portion sizes, listen to hunger cues, and practice mindful eating to support digestion and maintain a healthy weight.

· **Hydration:** Ensure adequate water intake throughout the day for proper hydration and overall health.

3. Mental and Emotional Wellness:

· **Stress Management:** Practice stress-relief techniques like meditation, deep breathing, or yoga to manage stress levels.

· **Positive Relationships:** Foster healthy relationships and social connections, which play a significant role in mental well-being.

· **Mental Stimulation:** Engage in activities that challenge the mind, such as puzzles, reading, learning new skills, or creative hobbies.

4. Quality Sleep:

· **Establish Sleep Routine:** Maintain consistent sleep schedules and create a conducive sleep environment for quality rest.

· **Sleep Hygiene:** Practice good sleep hygiene by avoiding screens before bedtime, creating a relaxing bedtime routine, and ensuring a comfortable sleep environment.

5. Self-Care Practices:

· **Prioritize "Me" Time:** Dedicate time for self-care activities that bring joy and relaxation, whether it's a hobby, bath, or time spent in nature.

· **Mindfulness and Gratitude:** Practice mindfulness and gratitude exercises to foster a positive outlook and reduce stress levels.

6. Professional Wellness:

· **Regular Check-ups:** Schedule routine health check-ups and screenings with healthcare providers to monitor overall health.

· **Seek Professional Support:** Never hesitate to seek professional help, whether it's from healthcare providers, counsellors, or therapists, when needed.

7. Environmental Wellness:

· **Healthy Environment:** Create a clean and organized living and work environment to reduce stress and promote well-being.

· **Eco-Friendly Choices:** Make environmentally conscious decisions in daily life to contribute positively to the environment and personal well-being.

8. Financial Wellness:

· **Budgeting and Planning:** Establish a budget and financial plan to manage finances and reduce financial stress.

· **Savings and Investments:** Prioritize savings and consider long-term financial goals and investments for future security.

9. Continuous Learning and Growth:

· **Lifelong Learning:** Engage in continuous learning, whether through courses, workshops, reading, or skill development, to stimulate mental growth and personal development.

· **Adaptability:** Embrace change, adaptability, and resilience in facing life's challenges and uncertainties.

10. Community Engagement and Contribution:

· **Volunteer Work:** Engage in community service or volunteer activities to foster a sense of purpose and connection with the community.

· **Support Networks:** Be part of or create support networks that promote mutual help and positive relationships.

11. Gratitude and Reflection:

· **Practice Gratitude:** Cultivate a habit of gratitude by acknowledging and appreciating the positives in life.

· **Reflection Time:** Set aside time for self-reflection to assess personal growth, values, and goals.

12. Digital Detox and Boundaries:

· **Mindful Technology Use:** Establish boundaries for screen time and practice digital detoxes to reduce stress and improve mental clarity.

· **Balance and Boundaries:** Maintain a healthy balance between technology use and offline activities for overall well-being.

Incorporating these habits and practices into daily life can significantly contribute to ongoing wellness, fostering a holistic approach that encompasses physical, mental, emotional, and social aspects of well-being.

CONCLUSION

Recap of Key Points

1. **Understanding Gut Health:** Exploring the intricacies of gut health, acknowledging its significance in overall well-being, and recognizing the gut-brain connection as a vital component of holistic health.

2. **Factors Influencing Gut Health:** Delving into the various factors affecting gut health, including diet, lifestyle, stress, sleep, and environmental elements, highlighting their roles in maintaining a balanced gut ecosystem.

3. **Nutrition and Gut-Friendly Practices:** Emphasizing the importance of a nutrient-rich diet, including probiotics, prebiotics, fiber, and gut-friendly foods while addressing foods that may negatively affect gut health.

4. **Supplements and Gut Health:** Discussing the role of supplements such as probiotics, prebiotics, digestive enzymes, and omega-3 fatty acids in supporting gut health, while stressing the importance of professional guidance and quality in supplement selection.

5. **Lifestyle Practices for Gut Health:** Highlighting the significance of holistic wellness beyond diet,

incorporating stress management, quality sleep, regular exercise, and other lifestyle practices to sustain optimal gut health.

6. Long-Term Habits for Ongoing Wellness: Encouraging the adoption of sustainable habits and practices encompassing physical, mental, emotional, and environmental wellness, ensuring a well-rounded approach to long-term well-being.

7. Reflecting on Personal Wellness: Encouraging readers to introspect, practice gratitude, seek continuous learning, engage in self-care, and establish healthy boundaries in the digital age for a balanced life.

8. Commitment to Ongoing Wellness: Inspiring readers to commit to ongoing wellness by incorporating these practices into daily life, embracing change, seeking support, and contributing positively to themselves and their communities.

9. The Journey Ahead: Acknowledging that the journey to optimal gut health and overall well-being is ongoing, requiring dedication, adaptability, and an active approach to sustaining a balanced lifestyle.

10. Seeking Professional Guidance: Reinforcing the importance of consulting health coach, healthcare professionals, registered dieticians, or counsellors for personalized guidance and support in maintaining gut health and overall wellness.

TO THE READERS

Encouragement for Implementing Gut Health Strategies

Dear Reader,

Congratulations on completing this journey through the intricate world of gut health! You've gained invaluable insights into nurturing your gut and fostering overall well-being. Now, as you stand at the threshold of implementing these strategies, here's a gentle push to embark on this transformative path:

1. **You're taking Control:** By delving into this Book, you've already taken the crucial first step towards understanding the pivotal role your gut plays in your overall health. Embrace this knowledge as empowerment to make positive changes.

2. **Start Small, Start Now:** An implementing gut health strategy doesn't require a complete overhaul overnight. Begin with small, manageable changes - a probiotic-rich snack, a mindful meal, or a short meditation session.

3. **Embrace Progress, Not Perfection:** Remember, it's progress that matters, not perfection. Every positive choice contributes to nurturing your gut health. Be patient and kind to yourself throughout this journey.

4. **Harness the Power of Habits:** Building habits takes time and consistency. Start by incorporating one new habit at a time, gradually integrating it into your routine until it becomes second nature.

5. **Create a Supportive Environment:** Surround yourself with encouragement. Share your goals with friends, family, or online communities. Engage in discussions, attend health workshops, online health coaching and seek motivation from like-minded individuals or health coach.

6. **Celebrate Small Victories:** Acknowledge and celebrate your achievements, no matter how small they may seem. Each step forward is a testament to your dedication and resilience.

7. **Adaptability Is Key:** Life brings changes and challenges. Embrace adaptability in your approach to gut health. Find solutions that fit your lifestyle, counsel with health coach and change strategies as needed.

8. **Listen to Your Body:** Your body communicates its needs. Pay attention to how it responds to different foods, habits, and environments. Your body's signals are valuable guides on your gut health journey.

9. **Seek Guidance and Support:** Never hesitate to seek guidance from health coach, healthcare professionals, dieticians, or wellness experts. Their

knowledge and guidance can offer invaluable support on your path to a healthier gut.

10. **Trust in Your Journey:** Embrace the journey toward a healthier gut with optimism and trust. Every step you take today contributes to a vibrant, thriving, and resilient you tomorrow.

Remember, the investment you make in your gut health today ripples into every aspect of your life—energizing your body, nurturing your mind, and empowering your spirit.

Take that first step. Implement these strategies with confidence and commitment. Your gut—and your entire being—will thank you for it.

Here's to a vibrant, nourished, and harmonious gut health journey ahead!

With Warm Regards,

Dr. Anuj Boruah

Closing Thoughts on Achieving Gut Harmony

Dear Reader,

As I conclude this insightful journey into the world of gut health, take a moment to reflect on the wealth of knowledge you've gained. The pursuit of gut harmony isn't just a destination; it's a transformative journey towards a healthier and more vibrant you.

1. **Embrace the Power of Harmony:** Your gut is a symphony - a delicate balance of diverse microbes, nourishing foods, and mindful practices. Embrace this harmony, nurturing it with care and intention.

2. **You Hold the Key:** You now possess a treasure trove of information and strategies to unlock the potential of your gut health. Your choices, habits, and daily practices are the keys that unlock this potential.

3. **Mind-Body Connection:** Recognize the intimate connection between your gut and overall well-being. As you nurture your gut, you're not just improving digestion; you're fostering vitality, mental clarity, and emotional balance.

4. **A Holistic Approach:** Gut harmony isn't solely about what you eat - it encompasses your entire lifestyle. It's the culmination of nourishing foods, mindful habits, stress management, quality sleep, and positive relationships.

5. **Consistency Is Key:** Remember, it's the consistent, day-by-day commitment that yields enduring results. Small, intentional steps taken each day accumulate into remarkable transformations.

6. **Honouring Your Progress:** Acknowledge and honour the progress you've made. Every meal choice, every moment of mindfulness, every step towards balance - all contribute to your journey.

7. **Be Kind to Yourself:** Embrace self-compassion. Understand that this journey isn't about perfection - it's about progress. Be gentle with yourself as you navigate this path to gut harmony.

8. **Trust the Process:** Trust in the wisdom of your body and the guidance you've gathered. Trust that each decision you make in favour of your gut health is a step towards vitality and wellness.

9. **Share Your Journey:** Inspire and empower others by sharing your journey towards gut harmony. Your experiences, challenges, and victories may resonate and guide someone else on their path.

10. **A New Beginning:** As you bid farewell to this Book, let it mark not an end but a new beginning- a chapter in your life where you embrace the power to nourish, heal, and thrive from within.

Remember, achieving gut harmony isn't a finish line - it's an ongoing commitment to yourself, your health, and your well-being. Embrace this journey with optimism, determination, and an unwavering belief in the transformative power of your choices.

Thank you for embarking on this journey with us. May your path to a holistic approach of gut health fill with vitality, balance, and a deep-rooted sense of well-being!

With Best Wishes,

Dr. Anuj Boruah

UNLOCK YOUR HEALTH POTENTIAL: WHY HEALTH COACHING MATTERS

Understanding Your Needs:

Health coaching isn't about a one-size-fits-all solution. It's personalized—tailored specifically to address your unique health challenges and goals.

Holistic Approach to Wellness:

Embrace a holistic approach that transcends just diet and exercise. It's about nurturing your mind, body, and spirit in unison—finding balance amidst life's chaos.

Accountability and Support:

In a world filled with distractions, a health coach becomes your accountability partner, offering unwavering support, guidance, and motivation every step of the way.

Customized Action Plans:

Say goodbye to generic advice! A health coach crafts personalized action plans, breaking down complex health goals into manageable, achievable steps.

Building Sustainable Habits:

It's not about quick fixes—it's about cultivating sustainable habits that seamlessly integrate into your daily life, fostering lasting health transformations.

Empowerment and Education:

Gain knowledge that empowers you to make informed decisions about your health. Understand the 'why' behind your actions, fostering long-term lifestyle changes.

Stress Management and Well-being:

In today's hustle, stress is inevitable. Learn strategies to manage stress, prioritize self-care, and enhance overall well-being amid a hectic lifestyle.

Continuous Support and Adaptability:

Your health journey evolves, and so does the coaching. Receive continuous support, adaptability, and recalibration as your needs and goals shift.

Ready to Transform Your Health? Connect on Telegram:
- Reach out on Telegram at https://t.me/hc_nhi to take the first step towards a vibrant, healthier you. Let's embark on a journey to unlock your health potential together!

ABOUT THE AUTHOR

Dr. Anuj Boruah, a certified health coach, nutritionist, homeopath, yoga trainer and multi-faceted holistic healer, wasn't always the embodiment of wellness. He sailed turbulent seas, battling his own health storms—struggling with digestive woes that disrupted the rhythm of his life.

Driven by a fervent desire to conquer these personal health hurdles, Dr. Anuj ventured into uncharted territories. He donned multiple hats—absorbing wisdom as a Reflexology Expert, Mastering the Art of Healing as a Reiki practitioner, and delving into the science of mind-body connection through NLP practices.

Through relentless experimentation and a thirst for unconventional solutions, Dr. Anuj unearthed a holistic approach. His amalgamation of ancient wisdom, modern science, and personal experience birthed a transformative method—changing not just his life but the lives of countless others.

His mission? To share this newfound wisdom, to pave a path of lasting wellness for those entangled in the web of everyday health struggles. Dr. Anuj stands as a beacon of hope, aiming to guide others toward a harmonious existence—free from the shackles of daily health battles.

www.ingramcontent.com/pod-product-compliance
Lightning Source LLC
Chambersburg PA
CBHW071601270726
48661CB00017B/338